LOW-SODIUM RENAL DIET PLAN

Delicious Recipes for Kidney Health

Dr Lily Morgan

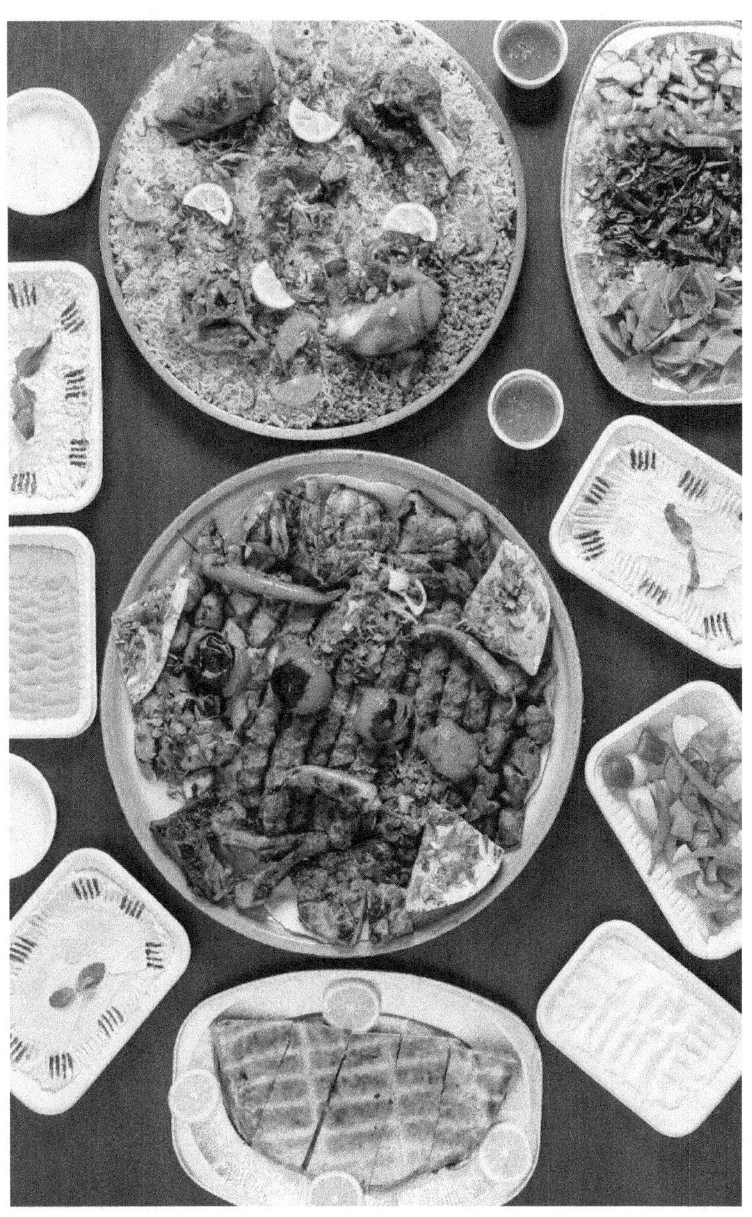

TABLE OF CONTENTS

Chapter 5: Snacks and Appetizers 61

INTRODUCTION

R enal health is a critical aspect of overall well-being, and one of the cornerstones of maintaining healthy kidneys is through a low-sodium renal diet. The kidneys play a vital role in filtering waste and excess fluids from the bloodstream, regulating blood pressure, and balancing essential electrolytes. However, when kidney function is compromised, as often occurs in chronic kidney disease, a carefully planned diet becomes instrumental in managing the condition and preserving renal function.

A low-sodium renal diet is specifically designed to reduce the intake of sodium, a mineral that can pose a challenge for kidney health. Sodium, commonly found in salt and various processed foods, has a direct impact on blood pressure. High blood pressure strains the delicate blood vessels in the kidneys, making it harder for them to function optimally. This is why limiting sodium intake is crucial.

But what does this mean in practical terms? A low-sodium renal diet involves minimizing processed and canned foods, which are notorious for their high sodium content. Instead, the focus is on whole, fresh foods like fruits, vegetables, lean proteins, and grains. These foods not only provide essential nutrients but also help in maintaining a healthy weight, another key aspect of kidney health.

Balancing nutrients in a low-sodium renal diet is a nuanced endeavor. It's not just about reducing sodium but also being mindful of other minerals and elements like phosphorus and potassium. In kidney disease, impaired kidneys struggle to regulate these minerals effectively. Hence, dietary choices need to address these concerns as well. For example, foods high in phosphorus, like dairy products and certain meats, should be limited, while potassium-rich foods such as bananas and oranges should be moderated.

This dietary approach isn't just about restriction; it's also about incorporating foods that support renal health. Reducing sodium and managing mineral intake is essential, but it's equally important to stay well-hydrated. Proper hydration helps in flushing out waste products and toxins from the body, relieving some of the stress on the kidneys.

In summary, understanding the importance of a low-sodium renal diet in renal health is pivotal for those with kidney disease or looking to prevent it. It's a proactive step toward preserving kidney function and overall well-being. By making thoughtful dietary choices, individuals can actively contribute to their kidney health, giving these vital organs the best chance to perform their crucial functions for years to come.

Chapter 1: 30-Day Meal Plan

Week 1

Day 1:

- Breakfast: Oatmeal with Fresh Berries
- Lunch: Lentil and Vegetable Soup
- Dinner: Grilled Lemon Herb Chicken
- Snack: Cucumber and Tomato Salad
- Dessert: Baked Apples with Cinnamon

Day 2:

- Breakfast: Scrambled Egg Whites with Spinach
- Lunch: Tuna Salad
- Dinner: Baked Tilapia with Lemon and Dill
- Snack: Guacamole with Baked Tortilla Chips
- Dessert: Chocolate Avocado Mousse

Day 3:

- Breakfast: Greek Yogurt Parfait
- Lunch: Quinoa Salad with Chickpeas
- Dinner: Beef and Broccoli Stir-Fry

- Snack: Fruit Kabobs

- Dessert: Berry Parfait

Day 4:

- Breakfast: Banana Almond Smoothie

- Lunch: Turkey and Avocado Wrap

- Dinner: Roasted Vegetables with Quinoa

- Snack: Greek Yogurt Dip with Veggies

- Dessert: Banana Ice Cream

Day 5:

- Breakfast: Sweet Potato and Apple Breakfast Hash

- Lunch: Spinach and Strawberry Salad

- Dinner: Lemon Garlic Shrimp

- Snack: Popcorn with Herbs

- Dessert: Rice Pudding

Day 6:

- Breakfast: Whole Wheat Pancakes with Blueberries

- Lunch: Baked Salmon with Asparagus

- Dinner: Vegetable Curry

- Snack: Cottage Cheese with Pineapple

- Dessert: Strawberry Shortcake

Day 7:

- Breakfast: Veggie Omelette
- Lunch: Black Bean and Corn Salad
- Dinner: Pork Tenderloin with Apples
- Snack: Celery and Peanut Butter
- Dessert: Peach and Blueberry Crisp

Week 2

Day 8:

- Breakfast: Avocado Toast
- Lunch: Vegetable and Barley Stew
- Dinner: Spaghetti Squash with Tomato Sauce
- Snack: Roasted Chickpeas
- Dessert: Chia Seed Chocolate Pudding

Day 9:

- Breakfast: Cinnamon Raisin Toast with Peanut Butter
- Lunch: Grilled Chicken Caesar Salad
- Dinner: Veggie and Tofu Stir-Fry

- Snack: Mini Caprese Skewers

- Dessert: Greek Yogurt with Honey

Day 10:

- Breakfast: Chia Seed Pudding

- Lunch: Spinach and Mushroom Quesadilla

- Dinner: Baked Cod with Herbs

- Snack: Mixed Nuts

- Dessert: Oatmeal Cookies

Day 11:

- Breakfast: Fruit Salad

- Lunch: Egg Salad

- Dinner: Turkey and Sweet Potato Chili

- Snack: Rice Cakes with Salsa

- Dessert: Mixed Berry Sorbet

Day 12:

- Breakfast: Breakfast Burrito

- Lunch: Hummus and Veggie Wrap

- Dinner: Cilantro Lime Rice with Black Beans

- Snack: Zucchini Chips

- Dessert: Angel Food Cake with Berries

Day 13:

- Breakfast: Rice Cakes with Cottage Cheese
- Lunch: Shrimp and Brown Rice
- Dinner: Lemon Rosemary Pork Chops
- Snack: Hummus and Pita Bread
- Dessert: Almond and Cherry Rice Pudding

Day 14:

- Breakfast: Breakfast Quinoa
- Lunch: Portobello Mushroom Burger
- Dinner: Mushroom and Spinach Stuffed Chicken
- Snack: Deviled Eggs
- Dessert: Fig and Walnut Bites

Week 3

Day 15:

- Breakfast: Spinach and Feta Frittata
- Lunch: Mushroom and Spinach Stuffed Chicken
- Dinner: Eggplant Parmesan
- Snack: Sliced Apples with Almond Butter

- Dessert: Lemon Sorbet

Day 16:

- Breakfast: Oatmeal with Fresh Berries
- Lunch: Lentil and Vegetable Soup
- Dinner: Grilled Lemon Herb Chicken
- Snack: Cucumber and Tomato Salad
- Dessert: Baked Apples with Cinnamon

Day 17:

- Breakfast: Scrambled Egg Whites with Spinach
- Lunch: Tuna Salad
- Dinner: Baked Tilapia with Lemon and Dill
- Snack: Guacamole with Baked Tortilla Chips
- Dessert: Chocolate Avocado Mousse

Day 18:

- Breakfast: Greek Yogurt Parfait
- Lunch: Quinoa Salad with Chickpeas
- Dinner: Beef and Broccoli Stir-Fry
- Snack: Fruit Kabobs
- Dessert: Berry Parfait

Day 19:

- Breakfast: Banana Almond Smoothie
- Lunch: Turkey and Avocado Wrap
- Dinner: Roasted Vegetables with Quinoa
- Snack: Greek Yogurt Dip with Veggies
- Dessert: Banana Ice Cream

Day 20:

- Breakfast: Sweet Potato and Apple Breakfast Hash
- Lunch: Spinach and Strawberry Salad
- Dinner: Lemon Garlic Shrimp
- Snack: Popcorn with Herbs
- Dessert: Rice Pudding

Day 21:

- Breakfast: Whole Wheat Pancakes with Blueberries
- Lunch: Baked Salmon with Asparagus
- Dinner: Vegetable Curry
- Snack: Cottage Cheese with Pineapple
- Dessert: Strawberry Shortcake

Week 4

Day 22:

- Breakfast: Veggie Omelette
- Lunch: Black Bean and Corn Salad
- Dinner: Pork Tenderloin with Apples
- Snack: Celery and Peanut Butter
- Dessert: Peach and Blueberry Crisp

Day 23:

- Breakfast: Avocado Toast
- Lunch: Vegetable and Barley Stew
- Dinner: Spaghetti Squash with Tomato Sauce
- Snack: Roasted Chickpeas
- Dessert: Chia Seed Chocolate Pudding

Day 24:

- Breakfast: Cinnamon Raisin Toast with Peanut Butter
- Lunch: Grilled Chicken Caesar Salad
- Dinner: Veggie and Tofu Stir-Fry
- Snack: Mini Caprese Skewers
- Dessert: Greek Yogurt with Honey

Day 25:

- Breakfast: Chia Seed Pudding
- Lunch: Spinach and Mushroom Quesadilla
- Dinner: Baked Cod with Herbs
- Snack: Mixed Nuts
- Dessert: Oatmeal Cookies

Day 26:

- Breakfast: Fruit Salad
- Lunch: Egg Salad
- Dinner: Turkey and Sweet Potato Chili
- Snack: Rice Cakes with Salsa
- Dessert: Mixed Berry Sorbet

Day 27:

- Breakfast: Breakfast Burrito
- Lunch: Hummus and Veggie Wrap
- Dinner: Cilantro Lime Rice with Black Beans
- Snack: Zucchini Chips
- Dessert: Angel Food Cake with Berries

Day 28:

- Breakfast: Rice Cakes with Cottage Cheese
- Lunch: Shrimp and Brown Rice
- Dinner: Lemon Rosemary Pork Chops
- Snack: Hummus and Pita Bread
- Dessert: Almond and Cherry Rice Pudding

Day 29:

- Breakfast: Breakfast Quinoa
- Lunch: Portobello Mushroom Burger
- Dinner: Mushroom and Spinach Stuffed Chicken
- Snack: Deviled Eggs
- Dessert: Fig and Walnut Bites

Day 30:

- Breakfast: Spinach and Feta Frittata
- Lunch: Mushroom and Spinach Stuffed Chicken
- Dinner: Eggplant Parmesan
- Snack: Sliced Apples with Almond Butter
- Dessert: Lemon Sorbet

You've now completed a full 30-day cycle of this low-sodium renal diet plan. Remember to adapt portion sizes and ingredients to your specific dietary needs.

Chapter 2: Breakfast Recipes

Energizing your morning with a wholesome breakfast is key to maintaining a healthy low-sodium renal diet. In this chapter, we present you with a diverse array of breakfast recipes that are not only delicious but also kidney-friendly. From warm oatmeal to refreshing fruit salads, you'll find options to suit your taste and dietary needs.

Oatmeal with Fresh Berries

Ingredients:

- 1/2 cup old-fashioned oats
- 1 cup unsweetened almond milk
- 1/2 cup fresh mixed berries (e.g., strawberries, blueberries, raspberries)
- 1 tablespoon honey (optional)
- 1/2 teaspoon cinnamon

Instructions:

1. In a saucepan, combine oats and almond milk.

2. Cook over medium heat, stirring occasionally, until the oatmeal thickens.

3. Transfer the oatmeal to a bowl and top with fresh berries.

4. Drizzle with honey and sprinkle cinnamon.

Scrambled Egg Whites with Spinach

Ingredients:

- 3 egg whites
- 1 cup fresh spinach leaves
- Salt and pepper to taste
- 1 teaspoon olive oil

Instructions:

1. Heat olive oil in a non-stick pan over medium heat.

2. Add spinach and sauté until wilted.

3. Whisk the egg whites with salt and pepper and pour them into the pan.

4. Stir occasionally until the eggs are cooked but still moist.

Greek Yogurt Parfait

Ingredients:

- 1 cup plain Greek yogurt
- 1/2 cup sliced strawberries
- 1/4 cup granola
- 1 tablespoon honey (optional)

Instructions:

1. In a glass or bowl, layer Greek yogurt, sliced strawberries, and granola.
2. Drizzle with honey for a touch of sweetness.

Banana Almond Smoothie

Ingredients:

- 1 ripe banana
- 1 cup unsweetened almond milk
- 2 tablespoons almond butter
- 1/2 teaspoon cinnamon
- Ice cubes (optional)

Instructions:

1. Place all ingredients in a blender.
2. Blend until smooth and creamy.

Sweet Potato and Apple Breakfast Hash

Ingredients:

- 1 small sweet potato, peeled and diced
- 1 apple, peeled and diced
- 1/2 teaspoon cinnamon
- 1/4 cup chopped walnuts
- 1 teaspoon olive oil

Instructions:

1. Heat olive oil in a skillet over medium heat.
2. Add sweet potato and cook until tender.
3. Add apple, cinnamon, and walnuts; cook for a few more minutes.

Whole Wheat Pancakes with Blueberries

Ingredients:

- 1/2 cup whole wheat flour
- 1/2 teaspoon baking powder
- 1/2 cup unsweetened almond milk
- 1/4 cup fresh blueberries
- 1 tablespoon honey (optional)

Instructions:

1. In a bowl, mix whole wheat flour and baking powder.
2. Gradually add almond milk, stirring until smooth.
3. Fold in blueberries.
4. Cook small pancakes on a non-stick skillet.
5. Drizzle with honey if desired.

Veggie Omelette

Ingredients:

- 2 eggs
- 1/4 cup diced bell peppers
- 1/4 cup diced onions

- 1/4 cup sliced mushrooms

- Salt and pepper to taste

- 1 teaspoon olive oil

Instructions:

1. Heat olive oil in a non-stick pan over medium heat.

2. Add bell peppers, onions, and mushrooms; sauté until tender.

3. Whisk eggs with salt and pepper, then pour them into the pan.

4. Cook until the eggs are set and slightly browned.

Avocado Toast

Ingredients:

- 1 slice whole wheat bread

- 1/2 ripe avocado

- Salt and pepper to taste

- A squeeze of fresh lemon juice

Instructions:

1. Toast the whole wheat bread.

2. Mash the avocado and spread it over the toast.

3. Season with salt, pepper, and a squeeze of lemon juice.

Cinnamon Raisin Toast with Peanut Butter

Ingredients:

- 1 slice cinnamon raisin bread
- 1 tablespoon natural peanut butter

Instructions:

1. Toast the cinnamon raisin bread.
2. Spread peanut butter evenly over the warm toast.

Chia Seed Pudding

Ingredients:

- 2 tablespoons chia seeds
- 1/2 cup unsweetened almond milk
- 1/2 teaspoon vanilla extract
- 1 tablespoon honey (optional)
- Fresh berries for topping

Instructions:

1. In a jar, combine chia seeds, almond milk, vanilla extract, and honey.
2. Stir well, then refrigerate overnight.
3. Top with fresh berries before serving.

Fruit Salad

Ingredients:

- 1 cup mixed fresh fruit (e.g., melon, grapes, kiwi, oranges)
- A squeeze of fresh lime juice

Instructions:

1. Chop the fresh fruit and combine in a bowl.
2. Squeeze lime juice over the fruit for extra flavor.

Breakfast Burrito

Ingredients:

- 1 whole wheat tortilla
- 2 scrambled egg whites
- 1/4 cup black beans

- 1/4 cup diced tomatoes
- 1/4 cup diced green peppers
- Salsa (low-sodium) for topping

Instructions:

1. Lay out the tortilla and add scrambled egg whites, black beans, tomatoes, and green peppers.
2. Roll up the tortilla, folding in the sides.
3. Top with salsa.

Rice Cakes with Cottage Cheese

Ingredients:

- 2 rice cakes
- 1/2 cup low-fat cottage cheese
- 1/4 cup sliced peaches
- A drizzle of honey

Instructions:

1. Spread cottage cheese on rice cakes.
2. Top with sliced peaches and a drizzle of honey.

Breakfast Quinoa

Ingredients:

- 1/2 cup cooked quinoa
- 1/4 cup chopped nuts (e.g., almonds, walnuts)
- 1/4 cup fresh mixed berries
- A drizzle of maple syrup

Instructions:

1. In a bowl, combine cooked quinoa, chopped nuts, and fresh berries.
2. Drizzle with maple syrup for sweetness.

Spinach and Feta Frittata

Ingredients:

- 3 eggs
- 1 cup fresh spinach
- 1/4 cup crumbled feta cheese
- Salt and pepper to taste

Instructions:

1. Preheat the oven to 350°F (175°C).

2. Whisk eggs with salt and pepper.

3. In an oven-safe skillet, sauté spinach until wilted.

4. Pour the egg mixture over the spinach, sprinkle with feta.

5. Bake for about 15 minutes until set.

Chapter 3: Lunch Recipes

When it comes to midday meals, variety is the spice of life, especially on a low-sodium renal diet. These lunch recipes offer a delightful range of flavors and ingredients, ensuring that your taste buds never get bored. From light salads to hearty wraps, there's something here for every palate.

Chicken and Vegetable Stir-Fry

Ingredients:

- 1 boneless, skinless chicken breast, thinly sliced
- 2 cups mixed vegetables (bell peppers, broccoli, carrots)
- Low-sodium stir-fry sauce
- 1 tablespoon olive oil
- Cooked brown rice

Instructions:

1. Heat olive oil in a pan over medium-high heat.
2. Add sliced chicken and stir-fry until cooked through.

3. Add mixed vegetables and stir-fry sauce; cook until vegetables are tender.

4. Serve over cooked brown rice.

Lentil and Vegetable Soup

Ingredients:

- 1 cup green or brown lentils
- 4 cups low-sodium vegetable broth
- 1 onion, chopped
- 2 carrots, diced
- 2 celery stalks, chopped
- Seasonings (bay leaf, thyme, pepper)
- Fresh parsley for garnish

Instructions:

1. In a large pot, sauté onions, carrots, and celery until tender.

2. Add lentils, vegetable broth, and seasonings.

3. Simmer for 25-30 minutes until lentils are tender.

4. Garnish with fresh parsley.

Tuna Salad

Ingredients:

- 1 can low-sodium tuna, drained
- 2 hard-boiled eggs, chopped
- 1/4 cup chopped celery
- 2 tablespoons low-fat mayonnaise
- 1 tablespoon Dijon mustard
- Salt-free seasoning

Instructions:

1. In a bowl, combine tuna, chopped eggs, and celery.
2. Stir in mayonnaise, Dijon mustard, and salt-free seasoning.
3. Mix well and chill before serving.

Quinoa Salad with Chickpeas

Ingredients:

- 1 cup cooked quinoa
- 1 can low-sodium chickpeas, drained
- Cherry tomatoes, halved
- Cucumber, diced

- Red onion, finely chopped

- Fresh parsley

- Olive oil and lemon juice for dressing

Instructions:

1. In a large bowl, combine quinoa, chickpeas, tomatoes, cucumber, and red onion.

2. Toss with fresh parsley and drizzle with olive oil and lemon juice.

Turkey and Avocado Wrap

Ingredients:

- Sliced turkey breast

- Whole wheat tortilla

- Avocado slices

- Lettuce

- Low-sodium mustard

Instructions:

1. Lay the tortilla flat and spread low-sodium mustard.

2. Add turkey slices, avocado, and lettuce.

3. Roll the tortilla and cut in half.

Spinach and Strawberry Salad

Ingredients:

- Fresh baby spinach
- Sliced strawberries
- Sliced almonds
- Balsamic vinaigrette dressing (low-sodium)

Instructions:

1. Toss fresh spinach and sliced strawberries in a salad bowl.
2. Sprinkle with sliced almonds for a crunchy texture.
3. Drizzle with low-sodium balsamic vinaigrette.

Baked Salmon with Asparagus

Ingredients:

- Salmon fillet
- Asparagus spears
- Lemon slices
- Olive oil
- Garlic powder
- Dill (fresh or dried)

Instructions:

1. Preheat the oven to 375°F (190°C).
2. Place salmon on a baking sheet and arrange asparagus around it.
3. Drizzle with olive oil, sprinkle garlic powder, and add lemon slices.
4. Bake for 15-20 minutes or until salmon flakes easily.
5. Garnish with dill.

Black Bean and Corn Salad

Ingredients:

- 1 can low-sodium black beans, drained
- Corn kernels (fresh or frozen, thawed)
- Red bell pepper, diced
- Red onion, finely chopped
- Cilantro
- Lime juice

Instructions:

1. Combine black beans, corn, red pepper, and red onion in a bowl.
2. Toss with fresh cilantro and lime juice.

Vegetable and Barley Stew

Ingredients:

- Pearl barley
- Low-sodium vegetable broth
- Mixed vegetables (carrots, peas, celery)
- Onion, chopped
- Garlic
- Bay leaf
- Herbs (thyme, rosemary)

Instructions:

1. In a large pot, sauté onion and garlic until fragrant.
2. Add pearl barley, mixed vegetables, vegetable broth, bay leaf, and herbs.
3. Simmer until barley is tender.

Grilled Chicken Caesar Salad

Ingredients:

- Grilled chicken breast
- Romaine lettuce
- Croutons (low-sodium)

- Caesar dressing (low-sodium)

Instructions:

1. Slice grilled chicken into strips.

2. Toss Romaine lettuce with croutons.

3. Drizzle with low-sodium Caesar dressing.

4. Top with grilled chicken.

Spinach and Mushroom Quesadilla

Ingredients:

- Whole wheat tortilla

- Spinach leaves

- Sliced mushrooms

- Low-sodium cheese

- Olive oil

Instructions:

1. In a pan, sauté spinach and mushrooms in olive oil until wilted.

2. Place tortilla in a skillet, add sautéed mixture and low-sodium cheese.

3. Cook until cheese melts, then fold the tortilla in half.

Egg Salad

Ingredients:

- Hard-boiled eggs, chopped
- Low-fat mayonnaise
- Dijon mustard
- Chopped celery
- Salt-free seasoning

Instructions:

1. Mix chopped eggs, mayonnaise, Dijon mustard, celery, and salt-free seasoning in a bowl.
2. Serve as a sandwich or on a bed of lettuce.

Hummus and Veggie Wrap

Ingredients:

- Whole wheat tortilla
- Hummus
- Sliced cucumber
- Sliced bell peppers
- Baby spinach

Instructions:

1. Spread a generous amount of hummus on a tortilla.
2. Add cucumber, bell peppers, and spinach.
3. Roll it up and slice in half.

Shrimp and Brown Rice

Ingredients:

- Cooked brown rice
- Shrimp, peeled and deveined
- Lemon juice
- Garlic powder
- Fresh parsley

Instructions:

1. Sauté shrimp with lemon juice and a sprinkle of garlic powder.
2. Serve over cooked brown rice and garnish with fresh parsley.

Portobello Mushroom Burger

Ingredients:

- Portobello mushroom caps
- Whole wheat bun
- Low-sodium barbecue sauce
- Sliced tomato
- Lettuce

Instructions:

1. Grill Portobello mushrooms, brushing with low-sodium barbecue sauce.

2. Place on a whole wheat bun, top with sliced tomato and lettuce.

Chapter 4: Dinner Recipes

When it comes to creating delicious, kidney-friendly dinners, this chapter offers an array of flavorful recipes designed with your health in mind. Each of these recipes is tailored to fit a low-sodium renal diet while ensuring that your taste buds remain delighted. From zesty Grilled Lemon Herb Chicken to comforting Turkey and Sweet Potato Chili, you'll find a diverse range of options to make dinnertime enjoyable and nutritious.

Grilled Lemon Herb Chicken

Ingredients:

- 4 boneless, skinless chicken breasts
- 2 lemons
- 2 cloves of garlic, minced
- 2 tablespoons fresh rosemary, chopped
- 1 tablespoon fresh thyme, chopped
- Salt and pepper to taste
- Olive oil

Instructions:

1. In a bowl, combine the juice and zest of one lemon, minced garlic, rosemary, thyme, salt, pepper, and a drizzle of olive oil to create a marinade.
2. Place the chicken breasts in a resealable bag, pour in the marinade, and seal the bag. Massage the marinade into the chicken.
3. Refrigerate for at least 30 minutes, allowing the flavors to meld.
4. Preheat your grill to medium-high heat.
5. Grill the chicken for about 6-8 minutes per side, or until it reaches an internal temperature of 165°F (74°C).
6. Serve with lemon wedges.

Baked Tilapia with Lemon and Dill

Ingredients:

- 4 tilapia fillets
- 2 lemons
- 2 tablespoons fresh dill, chopped
- Salt and pepper to taste
- Olive oil

Instructions:

1. Preheat your oven to 375°F (190°C).

2. Place the tilapia fillets on a baking sheet lined with parchment paper.

3. Squeeze the juice of one lemon over the fish, drizzle with olive oil, and sprinkle with chopped dill, salt, and pepper.

4. Slice the second lemon and place lemon slices on top of the fish.

5. Bake for 15-20 minutes or until the fish flakes easily with a fork.

Beef and Broccoli Stir-Fry

Ingredients:

- 1 pound lean beef, thinly sliced
- 2 cups broccoli florets
- 2 cloves of garlic, minced
- 1/4 cup low-sodium soy sauce
- 2 tablespoons honey
- 1 tablespoon cornstarch
- 1 tablespoon ginger, minced
- 2 tablespoons vegetable oil

- Cooked brown rice

Instructions:

1. In a bowl, whisk together soy sauce, honey, cornstarch, and ginger to make the sauce.
2. Heat 1 tablespoon of oil in a wok or large skillet over high heat.
3. Add the beef and stir-fry until browned, then remove from the pan.
4. Add the remaining oil to the pan, stir in garlic, and cook until fragrant.
5. Add broccoli and stir-fry for a few minutes.
6. Return the beef to the pan, pour in the sauce, and cook until it thickens.
7. Serve over brown rice.

Roasted Vegetables with Quinoa

Ingredients:

- 2 cups mixed vegetables (e.g., bell peppers, zucchini, carrots)
- 1 cup quinoa
- 2 cups vegetable broth

- 2 tablespoons olive oil

- Salt and pepper to taste

- Fresh herbs for garnish (e.g., parsley)

Instructions:

1. Preheat your oven to 400°F (200°C).

2. Chop the vegetables into bite-sized pieces and place them on a baking sheet.

3. Drizzle with olive oil, season with salt and pepper, and roast for about 20-25 minutes or until they're tender and slightly caramelized.

4. Rinse quinoa under cold water, then cook it in vegetable broth according to the package instructions.

5. Combine the cooked quinoa with the roasted vegetables and garnish with fresh herbs.

Lemon Garlic Shrimp

Ingredients:

- 1 pound large shrimp, peeled and deveined

- 3 cloves garlic, minced

- Zest and juice of 1 lemon

- 2 tablespoons fresh parsley, chopped
- Salt and pepper to taste
- Olive oil

Instructions:

1. Heat a pan over medium-high heat and add a drizzle of olive oil.
2. Add minced garlic and sauté for about 1 minute.
3. Add the shrimp, season with salt, pepper, lemon zest, and lemon juice.
4. Cook for about 2-3 minutes on each side until they turn pink.
5. Sprinkle with chopped parsley before serving.

Vegetable Curry

Ingredients:

- 2 cups mixed vegetables (e.g., cauliflower, bell peppers, peas)
- 1 can of low-sodium chickpeas, drained
- 1 can of coconut milk
- 2 tablespoons curry powder
- 1 tablespoon olive oil

- Salt to taste

- Cooked brown rice or quinoa

Instructions:

1. Heat olive oil in a large pan over medium heat.

2. Add mixed vegetables and sauté for a few minutes.

3. Stir in curry powder and cook for another minute.

4. Pour in the coconut milk and chickpeas.

5. Simmer until the vegetables are tender and the sauce thickens.

6. Season with salt and serve over brown rice or quinoa.

Pork Tenderloin with Apples

Ingredients:

- 1 pound pork tenderloin

- 2 apples, sliced

- 1 tablespoon olive oil

- 2 cloves garlic, minced

- 1/2 teaspoon ground cinnamon

- Salt and pepper to taste

Instructions:

1. Preheat your oven to 375°F (190°C).
2. Season the pork tenderloin with salt, pepper, and cinnamon.
3. In a pan, heat olive oil over medium-high heat.
4. Sear the pork on all sides until browned.
5. Transfer the pork to an oven-safe dish and surround it with the apple slices.
6. Roast for about 20-25 minutes or until the pork reaches an internal temperature of 145°F (63°C).

Spaghetti Squash with Tomato Sauce

Ingredients:

- 1 spaghetti squash
- 1 can of low-sodium tomato sauce
- 2 cloves garlic, minced
- 1 teaspoon dried basil
- 1 teaspoon dried oregano
- Olive oil
- Grated Parmesan cheese (optional)

Instructions:

1. Preheat your oven to 375°F (190°C).
2. Cut the spaghetti squash in half lengthwise and scoop out the seeds.
3. Drizzle with olive oil, season with salt and pepper, and place cut side down on a baking sheet.
4. Bake for 30-40 minutes or until the squash is tender.
5. In a saucepan, sauté minced garlic, then add tomato sauce and dried herbs.
6. Simmer for a few minutes.
7. Use a fork to scrape the cooked squash into "spaghetti" strands.
8. Top with tomato sauce and, if desired, sprinkle with Parmesan cheese.

Veggie and Tofu Stir-Fry

Ingredients:

- 1 block of firm tofu, cubed
- 2 cups mixed vegetables (e.g., bell peppers, broccoli, snap peas)
- 2 tablespoons low-sodium soy sauce
- 1 tablespoon honey

- 1 tablespoon cornstarch

- 1 teaspoon ginger, minced

- 2 tablespoons vegetable oil

- Cooked brown rice

Instructions:

1. In a bowl, whisk together soy sauce, honey, cornstarch, and ginger to create the sauce.
2. Heat 1 tablespoon of oil in a wok or large skillet over high heat.
3. Add tofu and stir-fry until golden brown.
4. Remove tofu from the pan.
5. Add the remaining oil to the pan, stir in mixed vegetables, and stir-fry for a few minutes.
6. Return the tofu to the pan, pour in the sauce, and cook until it thickens.
7. Serve over brown rice.

Baked Cod with Herbs

Ingredients:

- 4 cod fillets

- 2 tablespoons olive oil

- 1 tablespoon fresh herbs (e.g., thyme, rosemary), chopped
- 2 cloves garlic, minced
- Salt and pepper to taste
- Lemon wedges

Instructions:

1. Preheat your oven to 400°F (200°C).
2. Place the cod fillets on a baking sheet lined with parchment paper.
3. Drizzle with olive oil, sprinkle with herbs, minced garlic, salt, and pepper.
4. Bake for 15-20 minutes or until the fish flakes easily with a fork.
5. Serve with lemon wedges.

Turkey and Sweet Potato Chili

Ingredients:

- 1 pound ground turkey
- 2 sweet potatoes, diced
- 1 can of low-sodium black beans, drained
- 1 can of low-sodium diced tomatoes

- 1 onion, chopped
- 2 cloves garlic, minced
- 2 tablespoons chili powder
- Salt and pepper to taste

Instructions:

1. In a large pot, brown the ground turkey over medium heat.
2. Add chopped onions and minced garlic and sauté for a few minutes.
3. Stir in chili powder, salt, and pepper.
4. Add sweet potatoes, black beans, and diced tomatoes.
5. Simmer until the sweet potatoes are tender, stirring occasionally.

Cilantro Lime Rice with Black Beans

Ingredients:

- 1 cup brown rice
- 2 cups vegetable broth
- 1 can of low-sodium black beans, drained
- Zest and juice of 1 lime

- 1/4 cup fresh cilantro, chopped
- Salt and pepper to taste

Instructions:

1. Rinse the brown rice under cold water, then cook it in vegetable broth according to the package instructions.
2. Fluff the cooked rice with a fork.
3. Stir in black beans, lime zest, lime juice, chopped cilantro, salt, and pepper.

Lemon Rosemary Pork Chops

Ingredients:

- 4 boneless pork chops
- Zest and juice of 1 lemon
- 2 tablespoons fresh rosemary, chopped
- 2 cloves garlic, minced
- Salt and pepper to taste
- Olive oil

Instructions:

1. In a bowl, combine lemon zest, lemon juice, chopped rosemary, minced garlic, salt, pepper, and a drizzle of olive oil to create a marinade.

2. Place the pork chops in a resealable bag, pour in the marinade, and seal the bag. Massage the marinade into the pork.

3. Refrigerate for at least 30 minutes.

4. Heat a skillet over medium-high heat and cook the pork chops for about 4-5 minutes per side or until they reach an internal temperature of 145°F (63°C).

Mushroom and Spinach Stuffed Chicken

Ingredients:

- 4 boneless, skinless chicken breasts
- 2 cups mushrooms, chopped
- 2 cups fresh spinach
- 2 cloves garlic, minced
- 1/4 cup low-sodium chicken broth
- Salt and pepper to taste

- Olive oil

Instructions:

1. In a pan, heat olive oil over medium heat.
2. Sauté mushrooms, garlic, and spinach until they're soft.
3. Butterfly the chicken breasts and stuff them with the sautéed mixture.
4. Season with salt and pepper.
5. In the same pan, pour chicken broth and place the stuffed chicken breasts.
6. Cook for about 5-7 minutes per side or until the chicken is cooked through.

Eggplant Parmesan

Ingredients:

- 2 large eggplants, sliced
- 2 cups low-sodium tomato sauce
- 1 cup part-skim mozzarella cheese, shredded
- 1/2 cup Parmesan cheese, grated
- 2 tablespoons fresh basil, chopped
- Olive oil

- Salt and pepper to taste

Instructions:

1. Preheat your oven to 375°F (190°C).
2. In a pan, heat olive oil over medium heat.
3. Sauté eggplant slices until they're soft and golden brown.
4. In a baking dish, layer eggplant slices, tomato sauce, mozzarella cheese, Parmesan cheese, and basil.
5. Repeat the layers.
6. Bake for 30-35 minutes or until it's bubbly and the cheese is golden.

Chapter 5: Snacks and Appetizers

When it comes to snacks and appetizers for your low-sodium renal diet plan, you'll find plenty of delicious and kidney-friendly options. These snacks are not only packed with flavor but are also designed to support your renal health. Below, we've listed unique and tasty snack and appetizer recipes to keep your cravings in check while staying true to your dietary needs.

Cucumber and Tomato Salad

Ingredients:

- 1 cucumber, sliced
- 1 cup cherry tomatoes, halved
- 1/4 red onion, thinly sliced
- 2 tablespoons olive oil
- 1 tablespoon balsamic vinegar
- Fresh basil leaves for garnish
- Salt and pepper to taste

Instructions:

1. In a bowl, combine cucumber, cherry tomatoes, and red onion.
2. In a separate bowl, whisk together olive oil and balsamic vinegar.
3. Pour the dressing over the salad and toss gently.
4. Season with salt and pepper to taste.
5. Garnish with fresh basil leaves before serving.

Guacamole with Baked Tortilla Chips

Ingredients:

- 2 ripe avocados
- 1 tomato, diced
- 1/4 cup red onion, finely chopped
- 2 cloves garlic, minced
- 1 lime, juiced
- Salt and pepper to taste
- Baked tortilla chips for serving

Instructions:

1. Mash avocados in a bowl.
2. Add diced tomato, red onion, and minced garlic.
3. Squeeze lime juice over the mixture and stir.
4. Season with salt and pepper.
5. Serve with baked tortilla chips.

Fruit Kabobs

Ingredients:

- Assorted fresh fruit chunks (e.g., strawberries, melon, pineapple, grapes)
- Wooden skewers

Instructions:

1. Thread the fruit chunks onto the wooden skewers in any order you like.
2. Serve immediately as a colorful and refreshing snack.

Greek Yogurt Dip with Veggies

Ingredients:

- 1 cup Greek yogurt
- Assorted fresh veggies for dipping (e.g., carrots, celery, bell peppers)

Instructions:

1. Serve Greek yogurt as a creamy and protein-packed dip alongside fresh veggies.

Popcorn with Herbs

Ingredients:

- Plain air-popped popcorn
- Dried herbs of your choice (e.g., oregano, thyme, or rosemary)

Instructions:

1. Sprinkle your choice of dried herbs over air-popped popcorn for a savory and satisfying snack.

Cottage Cheese with Pineapple

Ingredients:

- Low-sodium cottage cheese
- Fresh pineapple chunks

Instructions:

1. Combine cottage cheese with fresh pineapple chunks for a sweet and savory treat.

Celery and Peanut Butter

Ingredients:

- Fresh celery sticks
- Low-sodium peanut butter

Instructions:

1. Spread low-sodium peanut butter on celery sticks for a crunchy and creamy snack.

Roasted Chickpeas

Ingredients:

- 1 can of chickpeas, drained and rinsed

- 1 tablespoon olive oil
- Salt, pepper, and your choice of seasoning (e.g., paprika, cumin)

Instructions:

1. Toss chickpeas in olive oil and your preferred seasoning.
2. Roast in the oven at 400°F (200°C) until crispy, about 30-40 minutes.
3. Let cool before serving.

Mini Caprese Skewers

Ingredients:

- Cherry tomatoes
- Fresh mozzarella balls
- Fresh basil leaves
- Balsamic glaze (optional)

Instructions:

1. Thread a cherry tomato, mozzarella ball, and basil leaf onto small skewers.
2. Drizzle with balsamic glaze if desired.

Mixed Nuts

Ingredients:

- A mixture of unsalted nuts (e.g., almonds, walnuts, cashews)

Instructions:

1. Enjoy a handful of mixed unsalted nuts for a satisfying and heart-healthy snack.

Rice Cakes with Salsa

Ingredients:

- Low-sodium rice cakes
- Low-sodium salsa

Instructions:

1. Top rice cakes with a spoonful of low-sodium salsa for a tasty and crunchy snack.

Zucchini Chips

Ingredients:

- Zucchini slices

- Olive oil

- Salt and pepper

Instructions:

1. Toss zucchini slices in olive oil and season with salt and pepper.

2. Bake in the oven at 425°F (220°C) until crispy, about 20-25 minutes.

Hummus and Pita Bread

Ingredients:

- Low-sodium hummus

- Whole wheat pita bread, cut into wedges

Instructions:

1. Use whole wheat pita bread as dippers for low-sodium hummus.

Deviled Eggs

Ingredients:

- Hard-boiled eggs

- Low-sodium mayonnaise

- Mustard

- Paprika

Instructions:

1. Slice hard-boiled eggs in half and remove yolks.

2. Mix yolks with low-sodium mayo, mustard, and a pinch of paprika.

3. Fill egg whites with the yolk mixture.

Sliced Apples with Almond Butter

Ingredients:

- Sliced apples
- Almond butter

Instructions:

1. Dip apple slices in almond butter for a crunchy and satisfying snack.

Chapter 6: Desserts

These dessert recipes are not only kidney-friendly but also delicious and satisfying. From warm and comforting classics to refreshing fruit-based treats, you'll find a dessert to satisfy your sweet tooth without compromising your renal health.

Baked Apples with Cinnamon

Ingredients:

- 2 apples (any variety)
- 1 teaspoon ground cinnamon
- 1 tablespoon brown sugar (optional)
- 1/4 cup chopped walnuts (optional)

Instructions:

1. Preheat your oven to 350°F (175°C).
2. Core the apples and cut off the tops.
3. Place them in an oven-safe dish.
4. Sprinkle cinnamon over the apples and add a touch of brown sugar if desired.

5. If you like some crunch, sprinkle chopped walnuts on top.

6. Bake for about 30 minutes until the apples are soft.

7. Serve warm, and enjoy your guilt-free dessert.

Chocolate Avocado Mousse

Ingredients:

- 2 ripe avocados
- 1/4 cup unsweetened cocoa powder
- 3 tablespoons honey
- 1 teaspoon vanilla extract

Instructions:

1. Scoop out the avocado flesh into a blender.

2. Add cocoa powder, honey, and vanilla extract.

3. Blend until it's smooth and creamy.

4. Refrigerate for a couple of hours to chill.

5. Spoon into small bowls, and indulge in a healthy chocolate treat.

Berry Parfait

Ingredients:

- 1 cup Greek yogurt
- 1/2 cup mixed berries (strawberries, blueberries, raspberries)
- 2 tablespoons honey
- 1/4 cup granola (low-sodium)

Instructions:

1. In a glass or bowl, layer Greek yogurt.
2. Add a layer of mixed berries.
3. Drizzle with honey.
4. Sprinkle with granola for some delightful crunch.
5. Repeat the layers.
6. Finish with a drizzle of honey on top.
7. Dive in with your spoon!

Banana Ice Cream

Ingredients:

- 2 ripe bananas, sliced and frozen
- 1 teaspoon vanilla extract

- 2 tablespoons almond milk (unsweetened)

Instructions:

1. In a food processor or blender, combine frozen banana slices, vanilla extract, and almond milk.
2. Blend until it reaches a creamy, ice-cream-like consistency.
3. Serve immediately or freeze for a firmer texture.
4. Enjoy a healthy and refreshing banana ice cream.

Rice Pudding

Ingredients:

- 1/2 cup Arborio rice
- 2 cups unsweetened almond milk
- 2 tablespoons honey
- 1 teaspoon vanilla extract
- 1/4 teaspoon ground cinnamon

Instructions:

1. In a saucepan, combine rice and almond milk.
2. Cook over low heat, stirring occasionally until the rice is tender and the mixture thickens.

3. Stir in honey, vanilla extract, and ground cinnamon.

4. Allow it to cool, then chill in the refrigerator.

5. Serve your creamy rice pudding.

Strawberry Shortcake

Ingredients:

- 2 whole-grain shortcakes
- 1 cup sliced fresh strawberries
- 1/2 cup Greek yogurt
- 1 tablespoon honey

Instructions:

1. Slice the shortcakes in half.

2. In a bowl, mix sliced strawberries with Greek yogurt.

3. Drizzle honey over the mixture and stir gently.

4. Spoon the strawberry mixture onto the shortcake bottoms.

5. Place the shortcake tops over the strawberries.

6. Enjoy a classic strawberry shortcake with a kidney-friendly twist.

Peach and Blueberry Crisp

Ingredients:

- 2 cups sliced peaches (fresh or frozen)
- 1 cup blueberries (fresh or frozen)
- 1/4 cup rolled oats
- 2 tablespoons almond flour
- 1 tablespoon honey
- 1/4 teaspoon ground cinnamon

Instructions:

1. Preheat your oven to 350°F (175°C).
2. In a baking dish, combine peaches and blueberries.
3. In a separate bowl, mix rolled oats, almond flour, honey, and ground cinnamon.
4. Sprinkle the oat mixture evenly over the fruit.
5. Bake for 25-30 minutes until the topping is golden brown.
6. Serve warm with a dollop of Greek yogurt if desired.

Chia Seed Chocolate Pudding

Ingredients:

- 2 tablespoons chia seeds
- 1 cup unsweetened almond milk
- 2 tablespoons unsweetened cocoa powder
- 1 tablespoon honey
- 1/2 teaspoon vanilla extract

Instructions:

1. In a bowl, combine chia seeds, almond milk, cocoa powder, honey, and vanilla extract.
2. Stir well and let it sit for a few hours or overnight to thicken.
3. Give it a good stir before serving.
4. Savor this delightful chocolate chia pudding.

Greek Yogurt with Honey

Ingredients:

- 1 cup Greek yogurt
- 2 tablespoons honey
- 1/4 cup mixed berries (optional)

Instructions:

1. In a bowl, combine Greek yogurt and honey.
2. Mix until well blended.
3. Top with mixed berries if desired.
4. This simple yet satisfying snack is ready to enjoy.

Oatmeal Cookies

Ingredients:

- 1 cup old-fashioned oats
- 2 ripe bananas, mashed
- 1/4 cup raisins
- 1/4 teaspoon ground cinnamon

Instructions:

1. Preheat your oven to 350°F (175°C).
2. In a bowl, combine oats, mashed bananas, raisins, and ground cinnamon.
3. Drop spoonfuls of the mixture onto a baking sheet.
4. Bake for 15-20 minutes until they're golden brown.
5. Let them cool and savor your homemade oatmeal cookies.

Mixed Berry Sorbet

Ingredients:

- 2 cups mixed frozen berries (strawberries, blueberries, raspberries)
- 2 tablespoons honey
- 1 tablespoon fresh lemon juice

Instructions:

1. Place the frozen mixed berries in a blender or food processor.
2. Add honey and fresh lemon juice.
3. Blend until smooth and creamy.
4. Transfer the sorbet to a container and freeze for an hour for a firmer texture.
5. Scoop out and enjoy a refreshing mixed berry sorbet.

Angel Food Cake with Berries

Ingredients:

- 1 slice of angel food cake
- 1/2 cup mixed fresh berries (strawberries, blueberries, raspberries)

- 2 tablespoons whipped topping (low-sodium)

Instructions:

1. Place the slice of angel food cake on a plate.
2. Top it with mixed fresh berries.
3. Add a dollop of low-sodium whipped topping.
4. Savor the light and airy sweetness of this dessert.

Almond and Cherry Rice Pudding

Ingredients:

- 1/2 cup cooked rice (preferably Arborio)
- 1/4 cup unsweetened almond milk
- 2 tablespoons chopped almonds
- 1/4 cup pitted and sliced cherries
- 1 tablespoon honey

Instructions:

1. In a bowl, combine cooked rice and unsweetened almond milk.
2. Stir in chopped almonds, sliced cherries, and honey.
3. Mix well and serve as a delightful rice pudding.

Fig and Walnut Bites

Ingredients:

- 4 dried figs
- 1/4 cup chopped walnuts
- 1 teaspoon honey
- 1/2 teaspoon ground cinnamon

Instructions:

1. Slice the dried figs in half.
2. In each fig half, stuff with chopped walnuts.
3. Drizzle honey over the figs and sprinkle ground cinnamon.
4. Enjoy these sweet and nutty fig and walnut bites.

Lemon Sorbet

Ingredients:

- 2 lemons, juiced
- 1/4 cup honey
- 1 cup water

Instructions:

1. In a saucepan, combine lemon juice, honey, and water.

2. Heat and stir until the mixture is well blended and heated through.

3. Allow it to cool, then chill in the freezer until partially frozen.

4. Once partially frozen, scrape the mixture with a fork to create a refreshing lemon sorbet.

5. Serve in a bowl or cup and savor the zesty sweetness.

Chapter 7: Smoothies

These smoothies are designed to not only tantalize your taste buds but also support your renal health journey. Packed with wholesome ingredients and vibrant flavors, these smoothies are perfect for a quick breakfast, a refreshing snack, or a post-workout pick-me-up.

Green Detox Smoothie

Ingredients:

- 1 cup fresh spinach leaves
- 1/2 cucumber, peeled and sliced
- 1 green apple, cored and diced
- 1 tablespoon fresh lemon juice
- 1/2 cup water
- Ice cubes (optional)

Instructions:

1. Place all the ingredients in a blender.
2. Blend until smooth.
3. Add ice cubes if desired.

4. Pour into a glass and enjoy.

Blueberry Banana Smoothie

Ingredients:

- 1/2 cup blueberries (fresh or frozen)
- 1 ripe banana
- 1/2 cup Greek yogurt
- 1/2 cup almond milk
- 1 tablespoon honey (optional)

Instructions:

1. Combine blueberries, banana, Greek yogurt, and almond milk in a blender.
2. Blend until creamy.
3. Sweeten with honey if desired.
4. Pour into a glass and serve.

Spinach and Pineapple Smoothie

Ingredients:

- 1 cup fresh spinach leaves
- 1/2 cup pineapple chunks (fresh or frozen)

- 1/2 cup coconut milk

- 1/2 cup water

- Ice cubes (optional)

Instructions:

1. Place spinach, pineapple, coconut milk, and water in a blender.
2. Blend until smooth.
3. Add ice cubes for a chill.
4. Pour into a glass and savor.

Mango Tango Smoothie

Ingredients:

- 1 ripe mango, peeled and diced

- 1/2 cup plain Greek yogurt

- 1/2 cup orange juice

- 1/2 cup water

- Ice cubes (optional)

Instructions:

1. Blend the mango, Greek yogurt, orange juice, and water until smooth.

2. Add ice cubes for a cooler texture.

3. Pour into a glass and revel in the tropical flavors.

Strawberry Kiwi Smoothie

Ingredients:

- 1 cup fresh strawberries
- 2 kiwis, peeled and sliced
- 1/2 cup vanilla almond milk
- 1/2 cup water

Instructions:

1. Combine strawberries, kiwi, almond milk, and water in a blender.

2. Blend until it's silky and pink.

3. Pour into a glass and transport your taste buds to paradise.

Papaya Paradise Smoothie

Ingredients:

- 1 cup papaya chunks
- 1/2 cup Greek yogurt

- 1/2 cup coconut water
- 1/2 cup ice cubes

Instructions:

1. Blend the papaya, Greek yogurt, coconut water, and ice cubes until it's creamy.
2. Pour into a glass and savor the tropical bliss.

Chocolate Peanut Butter Smoothie

Ingredients:

- 2 tablespoons unsweetened cocoa powder
- 2 tablespoons peanut butter
- 1 ripe banana
- 1/2 cup almond milk
- 1/2 cup Greek yogurt

Instructions:

1. Combine cocoa powder, peanut butter, banana, almond milk, and Greek yogurt in a blender.
2. Blend until it's rich and chocolatey.
3. Pour into a glass and indulge guilt-free.

Orange Creamsicle Smoothie

Ingredients:

- 1 orange, peeled and segmented
- 1/2 cup Greek yogurt
- 1/2 cup almond milk
- 1 tablespoon honey (optional)

Instructions:

1. Blend the orange segments, Greek yogurt, and almond milk until creamy.
2. Sweeten with honey if desired.
3. Pour into a glass and reminisce about the classic creamsicle.

Almond and Date Smoothie

Ingredients:

- 1/4 cup almonds
- 4 pitted dates
- 1/2 cup almond milk
- 1/2 cup Greek yogurt
- 1/2 cup water

Instructions:

1. Blend almonds, dates, almond milk, Greek yogurt, and water until smooth.
2. Pour into a glass and experience the nutty sweetness.

Peach Cobbler Smoothie

Ingredients:

- 1 cup sliced peaches (fresh or frozen)
- 1/2 cup oats
- 1/2 cup vanilla almond milk
- 1/2 cup water

Instructions:

1. Combine peaches, oats, almond milk, and water in a blender.
2. Blend until it's like a liquid peach cobbler.
3. Pour into a glass and relish the dessert-inspired treat.

Raspberry Coconut Smoothie

Ingredients:

- 1 cup raspberries (fresh or frozen)

- 1/2 cup coconut milk
- 1/2 cup Greek yogurt
- 1/2 cup water
- Ice cubes (optional)

Instructions:

1. Blend raspberries, coconut milk, Greek yogurt, and water until it's smooth.
2. Add ice cubes for extra chill.
3. Pour into a glass and savor the berry-coconut fusion.

Avocado and Spinach Smoothie

Ingredients:

- 1/2 avocado, peeled and pitted
- 1 cup fresh spinach leaves
- 1/2 cup almond milk
- 1/2 cup water

Instructions:

1. Combine avocado, spinach, almond milk, and water in a blender.
2. Blend until it's creamy and green.

3. Pour into a glass and benefit from the creamy richness of avocado.

Watermelon and Mint Smoothie

Ingredients:

- 2 cups fresh watermelon, seeded and cubed
- 5-6 fresh mint leaves
- 1/2 cup coconut water
- Ice cubes (optional)

Instructions:

1. Blend watermelon, mint leaves, coconut water, and ice cubes until it's refreshing and pink.
2. Pour into a glass and enjoy the hydrating taste of summer.

Cucumber and Kale Smoothie

Ingredients:

- 1/2 cucumber, peeled and sliced
- 1 cup fresh kale leaves
- 1/2 cup Greek yogurt

- 1/2 cup water

- Ice cubes (optional)

Instructions:

1. Place cucumber, kale, Greek yogurt, water, and ice cubes in a blender.

2. Blend until it's fresh and green.

3. Pour into a glass and embrace the greens.

Carrot and Ginger Smoothie

Ingredients:

- 1 cup carrots, peeled and chopped

- 1-inch piece of fresh ginger, peeled and minced

- 1/2 cup orange juice

- 1/2 cup almond milk

Instructions:

1. Blend carrots, ginger, orange juice, and almond milk until it's smooth and zesty.

2. Pour into a glass and enjoy the revitalizing combination.

CONCLUSION

In the final chapter of our low-sodium renal diet plan, we reach the culminating point of your journey toward better renal health. This conclusion is not merely an end but a beginning—a launching pad to maintaining the positive changes you've made in your diet and your overall well-being.

As we wrap up this guide, let's reflect on the key takeaways and considerations that will help you sustain your renal health for the long term.

1. **Consistency is Key:** The most important aspect of maintaining a low-sodium renal diet is consistency. Continue to follow the principles of reduced salt intake and balanced nutrition that you've learned throughout this plan.

2. **Regular Check-Ups:** Regular check-ups with your healthcare provider are crucial. They can monitor your kidney function and make adjustments to your diet or treatment plan as needed.

3. **Stay Hydrated:** Adequate hydration is essential for kidney health. Ensure you're drinking enough water while still adhering to your dietary restrictions.

4. **Listen to Your Body**: Pay attention to how your body responds to the foods you eat. If you notice any adverse reactions or changes in your condition, consult your healthcare provider.

5. **Physical Activity:** Incorporating regular physical activity into your routine can benefit your overall health. However, consult your healthcare provider to determine a suitable exercise plan that aligns with your renal condition.

6. **Support System:** Surround yourself with a supportive network of friends and family. They can encourage you on this journey and provide emotional support.

7. **Variety in Your Diet:** Maintain a varied diet to ensure you're getting a broad spectrum of nutrients. This can make your eating plan more enjoyable and sustainable.

8. **Keep a Positive Outlook:** A positive mindset can do wonders for your health. Embrace the changes

you've made and remain optimistic about your future.

In closing, remember that a low-sodium renal diet is not just a temporary fix; it's a lifestyle change that can lead to improved kidney health and an enhanced quality of life. Your journey to better renal health is a lifelong commitment, and with the knowledge and tools you've gained from this plan, you're well-equipped to embark on this path with confidence and determination. Here's to your continued well-being and a healthier, happier you!

www.ingramcontent.com/pod-product-compliance
Lightning Source LLC
Chambersburg PA
CBHW060950260726
48661CB00005B/1823